Resurgence

From Stroke to Life.

Author: Peter. T. Raven.

This is based on real events.

First of all, let me tell you a
little bit about

Myself and what this story is
all about.

My name is Peter. and I am
46årOld at the time of writing.

This story is about what happened

in my life and how it affects my everyday life at present.

Okay Then We Begin!

I take you back to the 21 July 2012 which

was the day when everything changed.

I am the father of four sons, two of which are resident

in Karlstad.

Firstly, I would like to mention that when this

took place, I was homeless and lived in

My car for several months.

So, 21 July, a very hot and sunny day in

lovely Karlstad and I had
spent an entire

week with my beautiful sons

In this beautiful day, me and
my sons had

 gone inline skating around
the city and along the

the water where there are
beautiful walkways to go on.

We had been and had coffee
at a café in the city center

and the clock began
approaching 17 o'clock in the
afternoon, so we decided to
go back

Then the boys would eat food
at that time.

The return trip went without incident, but I

began to feel strangely tired.

The boys would go in and eat the food and I said

I go to the Cape and putting me to rests,

A few hours so we hear of later.

We parted at 17.30 hours and I was driving and

parked at the Cape, put me in
the back seat and fell asleep.

When I woke up again had the
dark

presented themselves and the
time showed 22.45 hrs. and
my son

Had sent a text message to
me.

I tried to focus on what he
wrote but

had a little hard to decipher
what it was, but

managed to finally see that he
wondered what I did.

I tried to talk to him and
managed to get

off two text messages before I
noticed that my right arm fell
to the floor of my car.

I was amazed and first
thought that struck

me was that my shoulder had
fallen asleep in the half

Prone position I was in.

I lifted up my right arm again
and

Started a new text message to
my son.

Suddenly thump and my right
arm had once again landed on
the floor of the car.

I thought it was strange
because I did not

To the fallen down on the
floor again.

In the same moment I stared
at my phone

and SMS I would send to my
son included

just a bunch of letters, no
coherent at all.

It struck me as odd because I know

I typed text.

I felt I had to try to sit

me up and would drive down the right leg against

the floor in order to be able to do it, but what? Me right leg did not budge either!

Now I started to understand what was

Happening and I knew my time was getting very limited.

With one last effort, I called up my son.

I tried to tell him that they have to

send an ambulance
immediately because I have a
stroke.

My son was scared and
confused and left

the phone to his foster father
and I tried

repeat that I got a stroke and
needed a

ambulance immediately.

My son's foster father said to
me that they would

come and pick me up instead
because it

would go faster than it would
take for

The ambulance to reach me.

We put on and I knew they
were going to

me.

In the meantime, I was
waiting I thought much on

My life, it looked like images
in my mind.

Damn this cannot happen to
me I was thinking

at the same time that I was
sorry and fought

In order not to burn out.

I thought the time was
standing still, I felt dizzy

and faint, realized that I had
to get up

and get out of the car to the
fresh air,

While I was waiting for my
son and his foster father.

"I was really worried about
you when it came

thought you would die.

I been completely gone
because I never have been
through this before, but I
cried much and I panicked.

This is my son's own statements and they speak for themselves.

 With my last power I used left

arm and the left leg to sometimes lag,

Alternately pull myself out of the car and tried to best I could to set me upright against the car.

When I finally succeeded with
this huge

feat, to stand upright outside
the car and

wait for help, I felt a little
more alert, but

at the same time, I felt at that
time the facial paralysis

On the right side seriously.

I stood and wobbled a bit
back and forth

because of fatigue and
exhaustion, when I

Finally saw a car came driving
towards me.

Finally had my beloved son
come to the rescue.

He came rushing towards me,
scared and with the tears
flowing.

He tried to help me, but due
to

the right side of the body was
completely paralyzed became

I simply too heavy for a 16-year-old.

So his foster father drove his car

further, then walked up to me and took a

hug-on me, and lifted me into the back seat of his,

car and the ride to the hospital began.

This trip I never forget.

The body wanted to stop
breathing and pictures out of
my life

passed in Revue and in the
distance I heard someone

scream that I have to stay
awake and I have to talk all
the time.

I could in my condition not
determine who was yelling or
why.

My only thought was that I
must survive at any price.

When we finally arrived at the
emergency intake on

Karlstad's hospital staff stood
and waited for us.

 I was immediately
transferred to an emergency

stretcher and was rolled in for treatment.

During the first day I had time with two skull

x-ray and clot-busting agents introduced

Intravenously for an hour's time.

The first day was brought I
was woke up every 15th
minutes

For blood pressure and blood
sugar shooting and each

time I got to speak with the
staff so they saw that

I was contactable.

After this gruesome first day I felt

me as a total package because I had not

slept, several blood tests and

Medical examinations.

The only thing I could think of was my kids

And that I must live for their sake.

So I decided to fight.

On my 3rd day I had stabilized so that

they could move me by taxi to Karlskoga

Hospital and checking on Department 1A which

Is a pure stroke ward.

There it became more skull x-ray.

I had to spend the first night in

monitoring and blood pressure shooting day two,

revealed staff to the two scull x-ray

from Karlstad not shown any
results and not the one made
in Karlskoga.

This puzzled the doctors and
the

decided that a magnet x-ray
was only

option that could reveal
where this

cerebral infarction started.

Said and done, in the evening,
I was brought

to magnetic camera which is
like a big

Tin drum which you go into
on a bunk.

This monster will check
through your brain with

a variety of methods including

High frequency sounds.

After such an inquiry, it feels
like

the brain was left in the
machine sounds

Spinning around in my head
the rest of the day.

On rounds day after the
doctor wanted to speak with
me.

He explained that they found
the plug/

attack and according to the
doctor he could see on,

The pictures that I was big
smoker ha-ha.

Why I find it funny?

Well because I never smoked
more than five cigarettes per
day ever.

But after reading a lot about
stroke on the internet

 so I too realized that smoking
is actually a killing factor.

So I decided to quit smoking.

I can't cross stop but I can
stair

Down to 4 a day to begin
with.

After these tours with various
tests

I thought I finally come to the
stage

I would take it easy and
collect me.

It turned out to be completely
wrong!

Now it was time for a new
poll and

This time it was about test

Of the neck by means of x-
rays.

Back to the couch and then
lying completely still

so the nurse slowly and carefully, could

examine every millimeter of the neck muscles

and blood circulation.

This study is to see if.

There is constriction of the blood vessels or on the breathing.

There is a risk that muscles become swollen and causes

Problems with food or
breathing.

It turned out to be all right.

"Nice" so now at last I get to

Room and rest, I thought.

But now had second thoughts
about health care

the situation.

Now it was time for sick
gymnasts to come

into the picture!

These people present
themselves in a very

friendly and nice way and
declare that they

Will help me to get started
with my training.

I should add that I myself
worked in the medic line of
work when Younger.

medic care and in particular
with orthopedics and

Psychiatry.

So my gymnasts asked me to
go with them

down to the gymnastics to try
out a

wheelchair and a crutch that
will be

My companion on the road.

We started my work out that
included that

get up on the legs and
touching on both the legs.

Also included is facial
gymnastics in scheduling.

For the first time since the
stroke, I should now

try to stand on both legs,
which is a terrible effort.

Trying to drive me in to the
rail system which is a steel

construction with two rails
and plates

Hold them together at the
bottom.

I try to stand still but the body
would fall to the right!

 I try to concentrate, try to
get

balance in the body and
manages to stand still

without knowing that I would
fall what happiness!

My sick gymnasts watching
me, smiling and

Call on me to take a step
forward.

I stare at them and they nod
and say "

Come on you can do it".

I grip the left railing hard and
staring

down on my right foot and try
to get it to take a step
forward.

Watching and sends the signal
to the foot and leg but
nothing happens!

The staff told me to start with
the left

feet, which would mean that I
am forced

Stressing the right leg to be
able to move forward the left.

Jeez, man becomes fearful
and hesitant but I

Tell me that I can do it.

With determined my starts I
move the weight

to the right leg and know the
importance of the hip

And thighs on the right side,
but dare I?

 I move quickly forward with
left foot, regain

balance and feel really proud.

I managed to distribute the weight, the staff will be

And waiting and I ask what they are waiting for?

They respond and now do the same thing with right leg!

But how then? I thought to myself

But staring down on the leg
and foot and

really tried to force a motion
of any kind.

I stood for a long time, a very
long time and tried to

forcing my foot or leg to move
forward

but nothing happened!

But all of a sudden!

Oh the leg moves forward,
actually very slow

And trailing but it is actually
moving forward!

What a great feeling.

I get the legs next to each
other again and

the staff says "very good job"
and I feel so proud.

The staff tells me to put me in

The wheelchair again because
it may be enough for today.

I get help from staff to the
Division.

We end with evening snacks
or make up to

every day Monday through
Friday should I work out two

hours to get as much
movement in

My arm and my leg as
possible.

The following days along the
same pattern and

the leg begins to move more
every day

and things are going better
and better to go forward

With the help of the needles.

When will the next mortal
blow from the staff.

Today P, try to go with the
help of a crutch!

I thought ' help, how the hell
should I succeed with

This? ", but at the same time,
I saw it as a challenge.

Of course I have to learn to
walk with a crutch!

I got a crutch as they
adjusted to the right length

and was told to go on me,
which I did.

I was fading a bit before I got

body in balance.

I tentatively moved up the left
foot and

Then I tried to follow suit with
the right leg.

Then suddenly it happened
that did not happen, I got

fell head over heels to the
right and landed in a pile on

the floor.

The staff rushed out to check
on if I injured myself.

They wanted to help me up
but I shouted ' no '.

I said I can get up myself and
did everything

I could come up with to take
me up again,

But I managed to not,
unfortunately.

So the staff helped me up in
the wheelchair again

, which is defeat!

 This made me downright
pissed.

My body is so strong, not
even go

forward with a crutch!

The staff was trying to tell me
to calm but I

replied only that I want them
to help me

to practice to get up from
lying down

Position on the floor itself.

If it happens once, it can happen more was my train of thought.

They promised to begin the exercise the same

Afternoon and so was the case.

Lying on the floor, on the
right side, not

Neither the movement nor
sensation.

Do like this: with the left arm
push yourself up in

Sitting position, try to get
balance.

When you can sit without
falling back, fold

right leg toward the left so you get into

tailors position, then try to fold

the left leg so that you can get up on left knee.

 With the left knee to the floor to take the support of the left

arm and try also to get up on it

right knee "absolutely not easy I know".

Now with the help of the left leg and left arm

push yourself up to a Chair or wheelchair, and you

have now managed to get up off the floor at your own care.

After this day, I was firmly determined I

To go and I won't fall any
more time!

The following days I struggled
as a possessed and

managed to get the legs and
feet more and more but

noticed another strange thing
with

Right foot.

I knew neither the toes or
heel and foot wanted

Does not come with wiggle
position in points either.

Very odd.

Spoke with the staff about
this phenomenon and the

would send referral to
orthopedic technician

a foot frame that helps direct
the foot

Forward and also keeps it
firmly against the floor.

  Said and done, an
appointment with the
technician showed up

a few days later and I got to try out and

Jeez what a difference!

Staff had also ordered a brand new

Wheel chair for me which was my own and even a

brand new crutch.

Now started training seriously.

But a concern remained.

The arm, what about your
arm?

Could say as much to the arm
has been trained in

the extent of the leg and the
foot but

Unfortunately, without any
results.

There is very little sensation
in fingertips but that's all.

No movement at all but it
hangs more or

less there as ornament.

 So my priority is that you will
understand right

leg and foot.

Meanwhile, the Department
1a, I have trained

incessantly and had decent
time both with

crutch and behold, even
shorter distances without!

In section 1A in Karlskoga, I
was under the

more than 2.5 weeks, my days
consisted of training

and outdoor training for
exercise and strength

Every day the whole weeks.

I was released from the ward
1A

 8 August and I was moved to
a short-term

accommodation in Degerfors
municipality, which is

The end of the world really.

Wherever you are it is uphill
slopes and

sitting in a wheelchair, there
is no further arrangement

with slopes everywhere.

My training has continued
and consists at present

 of both the arm, hand, leg.

I go every day so much I just
can't be bothered

To be able to get to as good
time as possible.

Physical training of arm and
joints is to

Maintain the softness and
bending ability of all joints.

Today, on August 22 and it
will soon be

past five weeks ago since the
stroke and I

feel refreshed and alert and
ready for new

challenges.

This is the story to date, but

will keep writing down my
thoughts and

The progress continues to
occur.

Yes, today is Saturday and the
date is 25

August 2012.

What has happened since I
last wrote?

I'll try to be detailed and
explain

as much as I can so you
understand my

State of mind during this time.

My days usually start at
05.30-06.00

then they should cancel itself
out of bed with the help of

the left arm and left leg.

During the morning hours is
right

Page more or less unusable.

When I came up in a sitting position is

It's time to try to get up out of bed and get

the balance of the body to be able to

move to the wheelchair.

Once you have the balance
starts fine

balance between bed and
wheelchair with

small tentative steps and I
need to know after

Very carefully before I move
on the right leg.

This procedure must be
completed every morning so

It is routine.

I have to also look at your
right foot before I

moving the leg.

This is because feelings on the
heels and toes of

right foot doesn't work and as
we all know

control your toes the balance
of bone so this is a

very important moment.

When I finally have dragged
myself to

the wheelchair starts a last
trip to the bathroom

with toilet visits and more a difficult

task of the shower.

Shower is a pretty tricky task with one

Functioning arm and one good leg.

Equipment that is a must in a custom

bathrooms are as follows.

A requirement is handle by the toilet and in the

The shower and a shower stool as well.

Well, toilet bowl usually act as

undressing site before the
shower because it is

only place that is low enough,
so you

can reach all the way to the
floor to

remove both socks, pants and

Underwear.

To get from the toilet bowl to
the shower should

I use the crutch if it is
unsteady,

but I tend to move me but.

Thus the left foot forward,
then easily lug

Right foot, slowly but surely
into the shower corner

And drag for shower curtain.

Washing and further details
be omitted

Because it is individual for
each person.

To find their own way to
succeed in this

feat.

When we finished we
showered and dried out

reasonably dry, it's time to try

Start dressing themselves and
this

Item takes about an hour.

Sitting in a wheelchair, we
must begin by

try to get in the right arm in
the right sleeve of the
sweater

"which is not easy" because
the arm is completely useless

and without sensation.

 When successful, push in

the head of the shirt and
finally stops the

the left arm.

When this is done it starts a bit hard

Bit to get the shirt over the shoulder and back.

This subsection does not sound so complicated but bear in

given that you've just
showered and the body is
easy

moist.

Add to you no feeling on the
right side so

Therefore, any operation
should be done with the left
arm.

Try ourselves sometime so I
can give you the feeling of

How bloody awkward it can
be.

Well then follows the fun
element with

underwear and pants.

The principle is similar but we
must lift and

Drag a bit at a time, but in the
end it was also

fitted underwear and pants.

 Pooh!

Hard is it: but now there only

socks and shoes and the
mounts to the

as follows, while the sock in
his left hand and

open it with thumb and
forefinger wood the

Over the foot. First the right
and then the left.

That a boy, now remains only
the shoes to be dressed

for the day's activities.

When it comes to my shoes so
I have been learning

me one hand tighing.

This means that you get wood
if shoe lace then

To make a fast knot in one
end of the string.

End with attached wooden in
the upper

the left side of the shoe and
then you take the string
around the

the road to the last hole on
the right side and follow the

then just holes cross-as usual
the whole

the way up.

You can now begin to
assemble the shoe on the
foot.

the right foot and to me that
means a shoe and a

plastic strip down for the
foot's ability to control
matters.

One can easily get in the foot
and I pull for quite

hard for stability.

To be able to tie a knot with
one

hand pulling to as usual but at
top

overlap, stop a small loop in the

and then for you through another loop

Through the first and tighten.

Now I tied my shoes and is ready to

go out and meet the staff for today's first coffee.

After coffee and breakfast,
which I also Cook

self-rolling, I now turn to the
elevator too go

The top two floors to the
training room.

Yes, exercise.

Well then I'll tell you what I
do for that

bring back my body functions
in full,

Or those good things are
going to get them.

I always start my training
with the wheelchair

in front of a wide table in
front of me.

This is to be able to carry out
this morning's first task.

I begin by setting up the
damaged

the arm on the table with a
crocheted pot holder during
the hand.

Then I grabbed the right wrist
and pulls out right arm fully.

First straight ahead to the left
and right

side of the table and
stretching out my arm as
much as possible.

This step is repeated about
ten times.

Then it's time for the wrist
and hand with fingers.

Using the left hand tie each

I straighten out fingers to
maintain

The tenderness in all joints.

 After this pass, so it's time for

nerve stimulation which
occurs with a ball of

rubber, which has long tags
and

This wonderful ball does
wonders.

One wheel simply over arm
shoulder, hand.

First at the top then the
bottom for best effect.

Massage with the ball about 15minuter.

Now it's time for a little harder but

very important arm workout.

It performs I by two cuffs

With a piece of string between them.

String running across a small
wheel and is in my case

Attached at the top of a rib
frame.

This training equipment is
available with both silent

and elastic line, in my
required a silent line of

best muscle workout.

The elastic rope becomes way
too wobbly and

the risk of injury increases
significantly because no

 concrete movement is
obtained.

I range one cuff on right

arm and rolls into the
wheelchair with back first

to rib frame and grab then the
other

The cuff with the left hand.

Then just drag right arm
slowly

but surely against the ceiling
and the pressure really out

the arm in full and then
release it back

Slowly again and repeat 20 times.

After this arm therapy remain two

moment of my training.

The first is standard stair workouts, which

means go up a flight of stairs and down again

And charged to the right leg
as much as possible.

The final part of my daily

training involves regular
honest walk in a

Long hallway, four passes
roundtrip.

This training I told you now, I run

twice a day, seven days a week.

OK, a little more information about me as a person

is well aware that I'm going through the process with a

mother diagnosed with terminal cancer and

This also affects my
consciousness, but this

make me stronger and make
me fight even harder.

Then can I mention that even
the housing question

up for grabs right now and
need to be resolved before
last August.

So some stuff also happens
around that

affect me mentally and
physically, but I

do not allow myself to feel
pain or

grief, because they are
destructive forces and that

I can't afford.

To conclude with writing this

 time, I can say that my time
has been

better and Lo and behold, but
yesterday the 24

August started two fingers on
my right hand

being able to move!

Sure it's not much but they move!

The arm is not dead after all, you can understand how

great this is?

This is what I can tell you today and I

will be back with more news when some time passed.

Today is 27/8.

Has been in the hospital most
of the day for

an evaluation and first day at

day rehabilitation.

Evaluation means that they
look to the

improvements you had time
to do and what you

still having problems with.

 In my case is the situation
like this:

My arm has no function in
above or below

arm, the positive aspect of
the arm is to feel

In the skin come back a little
bit.

Not a feather-light touch, but
with slight pressure

I feel throughout the length and

Your fingers can now move in the hugging motion.

All fingers except the thumb who persist in to play dead.

The current balance is very good and without any fall trends.

Tested like this: Stand feet
together and stand
completely upright.

Then, close your eyes and
you'll try

maintain balance even with
your eyes closed

which is not easy.

For me, I can keep the
balance for about ten

seconds before I get wobbly
and get cases

trends due to stroke.

 After this step, it is high time that

check the strength of the body after intense

training for 14 days.

First up is to see how my time has changed

from the beginning it was my time a little bit trailing

And the body leaned very
right.

But the results after my
training is a non

trailing gait, and far less
inclination

Of the body during the walk.

Therefore, summary time and strength

Training has given good results.

In addition to the actual strength part of

Leg, arm and chest muscles.

We start with the bone: my
leg, straightened out

as good as the left with some

Effort, the physiotherapist
was received with slight
pressure.

According to her are leg much
stronger than

in the past, and she has some trouble pressing

received when I press the leg up.

The next step is to squeeze your leg back so

much as you can, the physiotherapist retrying

keep and this particular moment is very exhausting for me.

This is because the muscles
that will be

push backwards does not
work quite as they should,

so the power is much lower
but however

Stronger than for 14 days ago.

Foot on the right side has
from the beginning been a

problems, and not much
change has taken place

there.

I have the strength to push
forward, but some muscles

lack the power to pull the foot
up against

the body.

So summary is: movement
ability in

the leg has improved a great
deal which is

very positive.

Movement of the foot is,
unfortunately, in large

Unchanged which is not a
good sign.

Now I ordered to go and put
me on

 back at the brits in the
gymnastics Hall, they want to
look

a little more on body balance.

Thus lying on your back, pull
up both legs

To the bent knee position and
both feet down at bench.

Assemble the legs and bend
both legs first to

right and then to the left side,
do this

item two times.

Then, lift your pelvis/buttocks
from bunk

with leg help twice, at this

moment I am weaker on the
right side, so the cod-end

Get a little unsteady initially.

But I manage nonetheless
perform two lift.

Now to the final examination
of my

Evaluation and for my right
foot.

I will be asked to remove the
shoe and foot frame

from the leg as I do, the test
starts with

the staff's help, I will now
push the foot

Down as much as I can.

Which leads to a downward movement with about five

centimeters.

Now, I am told to pull the foot up, which

Do not give any movement at all.

This is because the muscles that

controls the tilt ability are not
Working at all.

She now wants me to touch
the toes on my

Right foot which does not
lead to anything at all.

Summary is that the foot is
and probably

remains partially paralyzed
because there is no sense of
touch

see either the heel or toes,
and there is also

No power to perform the tilt feature.

Another test sequence was carried out concerning

the stubborn right arm and went like this:

The first step is to add an unknown subject

in the right hand Palm and you

close my eyes throughout the
test, with the help of

the left hand should you now
identify the object.

Known throughout the hand
and can

way to produce if the subject
is cold or warm

the form in which it has
roughly and on surface

is hard or soft, this is no easy
task

because I have almost no
sensation at all inside

the hand.

Further in the arm test is so I
try to straighten out

my arm with only muscle
power, which becomes

a big fiasco because no force,
see

neither over or forearm.

Summary is that the hand can move four

fingers "very good" over and under arm

have no power "more training required" axis

and shoulder have power and
are strong which is

very good.

This is the assessment that is
the basis

for further referral to the
regional hospital in Orebro.

Now over to day
rehabilitation and the

includes largely just to hang
out with you people.

 others in the same situation
and coffee and a little more

training.

Well today, it is the 23rd
September 2012.

Yes, it's been a while since I
wrote something as a

Some changes have taken place to date.

Then out from short time accommodation in

Degerfors, I have now lived with my brother in

A few weeks ' time.

What has changed?

Since I wrote the last
movement in both hand

and arm improved
significantly, the hand can
now touch all five fingers.

Movement is limited
unfortunately of aches and

Swelling in both hand and
wrist.

The wrist can bend up and
down max 5

times since the exhaustion
and cannot more.

Hand's fingers are capable
know of to squeeze

easy stuff around but not with
force enough to

clip or lift, the biggest concern is

However, letting go, then, straighten the fingers.

 On physical gymnastics, we have continued training

with both arm and leg along with

balance.

The training we do with arm is that I

lying on your back to lift the
arm from lying

to resting on the elbow, but
that neither

Wobble or fall back. "Trust me
this is

not an easy task!

When I finally, with the help
of the eyes

stabilized his arm in this
position, will now

the next challenge to from
elbow mode press

arm up towards the ceiling
and this my friends

Manage maybe once out of 10 attempts.

We see this as a very simple thing but

After a stroke, it is a very difficult

task, we know his arm and
shouting at the in

its interior to rise up against
the ceiling as it usually
ignores.

This is and feels very
frustrating but

is a very important part of the
exercise to regain

Control of your nerves and
muscles again.

If we manage to reach toward
the ceiling, it is

 an achievement unparalleled
to give absolutely everything

in order to do this.

Then follow further exercises,
with the arm in

Arm bow mode I'll now try to
tilt it

backward against the staff's
hand and touch at

and then back to the original
position

again, it goes with the
tenacity and strength but it

Eating away at the forces.

After this step remains a
further and

It is from the elbow position
let the arm

slowly sit down to the
stomach without falling

And then back to the original
position again.

These exercises will be
repeated as many times as

you drop, then if you drop out
these

exercises at home which also
improve on your own

mobility.

OK on to the leg.

Since I wrote last, some happened even at

This area my sensation has improved in both

leg and foot.

The leg has obviously become
more powerful and capable

by both stairs and longer
walks without

major problems with the help
of crutch when walking
further.

of course, but the balance
has become a little better and

Therefore, my time.

The continued training of the leg consists of

walking and standing on a balance cushion, a

balance cushion is a rubber cushion intended for

both feet filled with some sort
of jelly for

to be varied.

Standing on this balance
cushion do I now

try to stand completely still,
which is not easy with

given the reduced sensation
and balance

on the right side, but we have run this exercise

a few times now and I think at present to

It runs really good.

Another exercise on this pillow is to

Standing on this, I will now
close your eyes and

maintain balance and this is a
very

difficult moment because my
balance is much decreased

with eyes that do.

I close my eyes and try to
balance the

runs fine at first, then I know
of cases

the tendency to the right time
I stood on the pillow

 corresponds to ten seconds
and that's what I

pass now.

So as you probably already understand, this is a

I am very unhappy with the results but it

is unfortunately in the condition my balance is in

the State of play.

This exercise is part of a test
that is to

basis for further referral to
the central hospital in Orebro.

Another exercise includes the
following:

Seated in a regular Chair
without arm rests will

I drive myself without using
the fresh

arm and go a short trip turn
and go

back to the Chair and put me
softly without using

the hand.

This is done on time and my
time was last

34 seconds and is quite good
considering

I go slowly and have poor
balance not

true?

Oh well on to the next care
namely

 the foot.

It has been a major concern
since the start

But even here, the
improvements brought to the

position, previously I had no
sensation in either

toes or heel.

This has been improved in the
sense that I have

started feeling in right big toe
and the foot's wiggle

function has been greatly
improved and I can

Now bend the foot both
upwards and downwards.

Bending the foot upwards are
still not without

trouble and can't bend fully,
but it can

at least give in both up and
down

This is a great achievement!

Nursing gymnastics is now
tailored to me

improvements and emphasis
is put on the balance

and walking exercise.

I am also asked to cycle on
exercise

cycle on physical gymnastics
in order to maintain

both breathing and fitness of
the body and when

I bikes I usually use some sort of

glove for right hand, because it does not

Can grab and hold the handlebars by itself.

This glove looks like a long

leather glove with Velcro fastener on wrist

and in the front is what a long tongue, when

put your hand on the handle
bars is this

heavy and pulls over your
hand and thus becomes

hand completely encased in a
glove and you

stuck at the handlebars.

Pretty clever, in fact, if I may
say so

itself.

Well so far so good now to
the

refractory foot that always
has a tendency to

will rotate to the right, this is
solved by using

by an elastic band that strains
over your foot

And attached to the pedal of bike.

OK now we're ready to pedal away about ten

minutes by 1.5 Joule's load tends to be

fully sufficient training then you have trampled about

three kilometers.

Then as each day's training, I
usually step

out of the wheelchair and
have it in front of me to
support

for a hearty walk both on the
flat straight road

But even in crates to get
resistance.

In the evenings I usually go up
and down in

the stairs of my brother with
the help of

the handrail usually tries to go
up and down

the stairs three times and the
stairs is made up of 16

steps.

I also have all the training
schemes

health care written out to me
and used

On a daily basis to achieve
maximum results.

Tomorrow Monday, it's
another day on the

day rehabilitation that awaits
with more

training, on Tuesday following
a doctor's visit on

regional hospital in Orebro for
my final

evaluation and then emerges
from me

The ability to drive a car again and so on.

Time for my doctor's visit was postponed to

on September 29 on Friday because of

double booking for patients.

Yes, my friends today say the calendar to

the date is September 30,
2012 and I

 have completed my visit at
the doctor at

regional hospital in Orebro.

What emerged?

The doctor did a thorough
inspection of me

opportunities to be able to
move my leg, arm, foot

with the following results.

My leg can move relatively
well both forward

and backwards but have
distinct spasms at

load but also difficult to
maintain balance

By motion to the side.

This does, of course, my time and

the doctor does not believe this will change

significantly in the future.

My arm has been improved in terms of strength to

lift and hold it up for a long
while, no

much difference with regard
to squeeze and release

The grip on a mug or a pen.

When you try to grab a mug I
get strong

pain in the wrist and this
makes it impossible

to try to keep and draw my
hand than.

 less to grab the mug, this
depends on the

weakening in both wrist and
to the muscles

has thinned out considerably.

According to the doctor, this
will be coached

up to a certain degree but will
probably

Never be really good again.

My right foot Yes, it has been
a

concern for himself and now
it can be said that the

works fine after the
conditions I have

for it, the foot is able to bend
both up and

down to constrained modes,
turning the foot in

Lateral work to the left but
not to the right.

Contributing to the foot
would like to turn to the

right in the time ahead, so my
goal should be to

try to keep your foot straight
at the time and not over

strain at normal walk.

Regarding the sensation in the
foot is missing it in right

page on the above page, and
almost all of the

The underside of the foot.

These mobility problems that
remain can be difficult

If not impossible to work out,
but I get

Learn to live with them during
the time the

 the body tries to heal which
is a

process that can take years to
achieve.

Additional information
resulting from

doctor's visit was that my
facial paralysis

not lost but are still present
and causes

Some speech problems, and
according to the doctor reads

This clinical picture aphasia
which is

speech impairment.

Then it emerged that my eyes
do not

keep up with reaction in
following

a finger as the doctor holds
up in front of you

and move sideways and up
and down, my eyes

React but not fast enough.

So with these factors added
to my

current situation does not
directly cause

easier to deal with but I have no

Choice but to keep fighting.

Within 14 days, I get further information from

Orebro if I will be inserted on the

Rehabilitation Department or if I won't.

will have to take a taxi
between three days per

week, this is the information I
have included

and also you readers as I write

down the information I myself
is notified.

This and my further fortunes
do I tell at

a later time.

For you people out there who
doubted me

ability to recover me so sorry I
am

stronger than you thought,
and for those of you who
think

I set high goals, I can only say

I always aim for the stars and I
will reach my goals.

Finally, a Word to your others
in the same situation: aim for
the stars and always continue
to fight large

Hugs to you all.

A final thank you to the
following wards

with Staff.

Central Hospital in Karlstad
emergency room/stroke

Ward

Karlskoga hospital Ward 1A

Västergården in Degerfors.

Nursing gymnastics at
Karlskoga hospital

A big thank you to all of you, without you I would not be here.

Where I am today I bow deeply to you all.

Thanks to you readers and who knows maybe we get in touch again.

With a warm greeting.

P. Raven.